LYMPHEDEMA DIET COOKBOOK FOR SENIORS

Empowering Strategies for Wellness: Incorporating Nutrient-Rich Foods, Vital Vitamins, Essential Minerals, and Beneficial Supplements Alongside Therapeutic Exercise Routines.

Ralph Hannah

DISCLAIMER

This publication is designed to provide competent and reliable information regarding the subject covered. However, the views expressed in this publication are those of the author alone, and should not be taken as expert instruction or professional advice. The reader is responsible for his or her actions. The author hereby disclaims any responsibility or liability whatsoever that is incurred from the use or application of the contents of this publication by the purchaser of the reader. The purchaser or reader is hereby responsible for his or her actions.

TABLE OF CONTENTS

INTRODUCTION
UNDERSTANDING LYMPHEDEMA IN SENIORS

What is Lymphedema?

A chronic medical disorder called lymphedema is defined by an overabundance of lymphatic fluid that causes tissue alterations and swelling. As an essential part of the immune and circulatory systems, the lymphatic system is critical for removing toxins from the body and preserving fluid equilibrium. Usually, lymphedema develops when the lymphatic vessels are damaged or disrupted, preventing the lymphatic fluid from flowing normally.

Causes and Types:

Lymphedema can be classified into two main types: primary and secondary. *Primary lymphedema* is often genetically predisposed and arises from developmental abnormalities in the lymphatic system. On the other hand, *secondary lymphedema* is more prevalent and results from external factors such as surgery, radiation therapy, trauma, or infections that compromise the lymphatic pathways.

Symptoms:

Common symptoms of lymphedema include persistent swelling, particularly in the limbs, which may lead to discomfort, heaviness, and restricted range of motion. Additionally, individuals with lymphedema may experience skin changes, recurrent infections, and an increased susceptibility to injuries due to compromised tissue integrity.

Diagnosis:

Accurate diagnosis of lymphedema typically involves a thorough medical history, physical examination, and, in some cases, imaging studies such as lymphoscintigraphy. Early detection is crucial for effective management and preventing the progression of the condition.

Management and Treatment:

While lymphedema is a chronic condition without a cure, various management strategies can help control symptoms and improve the quality of life for affected individuals. Conservative approaches often include manual lymphatic drainage, compression therapy, exercise, and skincare. In more severe cases, surgical interventions may be considered.

Impact on Quality of Life:

Beyond the physical manifestations, lymphedema can significantly impact an individual's emotional well-being and daily functioning. Coping with the chronic nature of the condition, adapting to lifestyle modifications, and seeking ongoing support are integral components of a comprehensive approach to managing lymphedema.

Preventive Measures:

For individuals at risk of developing lymphedema, such as those undergoing cancer treatment, preventive measures include meticulous skin care, avoidance of trauma or injury, and engaging in appropriate exercise. Early intervention and adherence to prescribed therapies play a crucial role in minimizing the impact of lymphedema.

How Lymphedema Affects Seniors

For seniors, lymphedema—a chronic illness marked by a build-up of lymphatic fluid—can have particular consequences. An in-depth understanding of the effects of lymphedema on seniors is necessary due to the specific environment created by the aging process and possible concurrent health conditions.

1. **Increased Prevalence:**

   - The likelihood of developing lymphedema tends to increase with age, as the aging process may contribute to diminished lymphatic function and reduced tissue elasticity.

2. **Complications from Coexisting Conditions:**

   - Seniors often contend with various health conditions requiring medical interventions such as surgery or radiation, both of which are common triggers for secondary lymphedema. Coexisting conditions like heart disease or diabetes may exacerbate the challenges of managing lymphedema in older adults.

3. Impact on Mobility and Independence:

- Lymphedema-related swelling, particularly in the limbs, can hinder mobility and compromise independence for seniors. Reduced flexibility and increased risk of falls may result from the heaviness and discomfort associated with swollen limbs.

4. Skin Integrity and Infections:

- Aging skin is more susceptible to damage and infections, and seniors with lymphedema may face additional challenges in maintaining skin integrity. The compromised lymphatic system can make them more prone to cellulitis and other skin infections, necessitating diligent skin care.

5. Quality of Life Considerations:

- Lymphedema can have profound effects on the emotional and psychological well-being of seniors. Coping with a chronic condition, potential physical limitations, and changes in body image can impact their overall quality of life.

6. Adherence to Treatment:

- Seniors may face unique challenges in adhering to prescribed lymphedema management strategies. Factors such as cognitive decline, limited mobility, or financial constraints may impact their ability to consistently engage in recommended therapies like compression garments, exercise, or manual lymphatic drainage.

7. Preventive Measures for Aging Individuals:

- For seniors at risk of developing lymphedema, proactive measures become pivotal. Strategies such as promoting overall wellness, emphasizing skin care, and incorporating gentle exercises into daily routines can contribute to preventing the onset or progression of lymphedema.

8. Collaboration with Healthcare Professionals:

- Effective management of lymphedema in seniors requires a collaborative approach involving healthcare professionals, caregivers, and the individuals themselves. Regular monitoring, tailored treatment plans, and education play critical roles in optimizing outcomes.

THE BASICS OF A LYMPHEDEMA-FRIENDLY DIET

Key Principles of a Lymphedema Die

The chronic illness known as lymphedema, which is characterized by a build-up of lymphatic fluid, requires a careful and specific diet. An intelligent food plan for lymphedema concentrates on controlling fluid balance, lowering inflammation, and enhancing general health.

1. Balanced Nutrition:

- A lymphedema-friendly diet emphasizes a balanced intake of macronutrients (carbohydrates, proteins, and fats) and micronutrients (vitamins and minerals). A diverse and nutrient-rich diet supports overall health and aids in managing the condition.

2. Controlled Sodium Intake:

- Excessive sodium can contribute to fluid retention, exacerbating lymphedema symptoms. The diet should aim to limit sodium intake by avoiding processed foods, using herbs and spices for flavor, and choosing fresh, whole foods over packaged alternatives.

3. Adequate Hydration:

- While managing sodium is crucial, maintaining proper hydration is equally important. Ample water intake supports lymphatic function and helps flush toxins from the body. Individuals should aim for a well-balanced approach to hydration without excessive fluid intake.

4. Moderation in Protein Consumption:

- Protein is essential for tissue repair and overall health. However, excessive protein intake may contribute to fluid buildup. The diet should include moderate amounts of lean proteins, incorporating sources such as poultry, fish, legumes, and dairy.

5. Healthy Fats:

- Incorporating healthy fats, such as those found in avocados, nuts, seeds, and olive oil, supports overall well-being. These fats contribute to a balanced diet without compromising lymphatic function.

6. Emphasis on Whole Foods:

- Whole, unprocessed foods form the foundation of a lymphedema diet. Fresh fruits, vegetables, whole grains, and lean proteins provide essential nutrients while minimizing the intake of additives and preservatives.

7. Regular, Small Meals:

- Eating smaller, more frequent meals throughout the day helps manage blood sugar levels and reduces the burden on the lymphatic system. This approach promotes steady energy levels and aids in avoiding large fluid influxes.

8. Mindful Eating:

- Being mindful of eating habits, including chewing thoroughly and savoring meals, can contribute to better digestion and nutrient absorption. This principle emphasizes the importance of paying attention to the body's signals of hunger and satiety.

9. Individualized Approach:

- Every individual's response to foods may vary. An effective lymphedema diet takes into account personal preferences, cultural considerations, and any coexisting health conditions. Consulting with a healthcare professional or a registered dietitian can help tailor dietary recommendations to individual needs.

10. Gradual Changes and Monitoring:

- Implementing dietary changes gradually allows for better adaptation and observation of their impact. Regular monitoring of lymphedema symptoms, weight, and overall well-being helps individuals and healthcare professionals make informed adjustments to the diet plan.

Importance of Proper Nutrition for Seniors

An essential component of optimal health is proper nutrition, and as people age, the importance of this becomes more apparent. A well-balanced, nutrient-rich diet is especially beneficial to seniors because it is essential for preserving mental and physical health as well as avoiding and treating several age-related illnesses.

1. Maintenance of Physical Health:

- Adequate nutrition is fundamental for preserving muscle mass, bone density, and overall physical function in seniors. Essential nutrients, such as protein, calcium, and vitamin D, become paramount to sustain mobility, reduce the risk of fractures, and support the body's ability to recover from illnesses or injuries.

2. Disease Prevention and Management:

- Proper nutrition plays a pivotal role in preventing and managing chronic conditions commonly associated with aging, including cardiovascular diseases, diabetes, and osteoporosis. A diet rich in fruits, vegetables, whole grains, and lean proteins provides essential vitamins and minerals that contribute to overall cardiovascular health, blood sugar regulation, and bone density.

3. Immune System Support:

- Seniors often face a natural decline in immune function, making them more susceptible to infections and illnesses. A well-balanced diet, rich in vitamins and antioxidants from a variety of foods, helps support the immune system, enhancing the body's ability to fend off pathogens and recover more efficiently.

4. Cognitive Function and Mental Health:

- Nutrition has a direct impact on cognitive function and mental well-being. Omega-3 fatty acids, found in fish and nuts, antioxidants from fruits and vegetables, and B-vitamins contribute to brain health, potentially reducing the risk of cognitive decline and promoting emotional well-being.

5. Digestive Health:

- As the digestive system may experience changes with age, a diet high in fiber from fruits, vegetables, and whole grains aids in maintaining digestive health. Adequate hydration and fiber intake help prevent constipation and promote a healthy gut microbiome.

6. Energy and Nutrient Absorption:

- Seniors may experience changes in metabolism and nutrient absorption. A nutrient-dense diet ensures that essential vitamins and minerals are readily available, supporting energy levels and preventing nutritional deficiencies that can lead to fatigue and other health issues.

7. Maintaining Healthy Body Weight:

- Proper nutrition contributes to maintaining a healthy body weight, which is crucial for overall well-being. Seniors are at risk of unintentional weight loss, which can lead to muscle wasting and increased vulnerability to infections. A well-balanced diet helps regulate weight and supports healthy aging.

8. Hydration:

- Adequate hydration is a key aspect of proper nutrition for seniors. Dehydration can lead to a range of health issues, including dizziness, urinary tract infections, and impaired cognitive function. Seniors should pay attention to their fluid intake, especially in cases where thirst perception may be diminished.

9. Quality of Life and Independence:

- Proper nutrition is closely linked to maintaining a high quality of life and independence in older adults. A well-nourished senior is more likely to have the strength, vitality, and mental acuity needed to engage in daily activities, social interactions, and hobbies.

SENIORS AND HYDRATION

The Role of Hydration in Managing Lymphedema

Hydration is one underappreciated but vital component of the complex strategy used to control lymphedema. Maintaining adequate hydration is essential for assisting the lymphatic system, preventing fluid buildup, and improving general health in lymphedema patients.

1. **Lymphatic System Function:**

   - The lymphatic system, a network of vessels, nodes, and organs, is responsible for maintaining fluid balance, filtering toxins, and supporting the immune system. Hydration is essential for the optimal function of this intricate system, allowing for the efficient transport of lymphatic fluid throughout the body.

2. **Fluid Dynamics and Hydration:**

   - Adequate hydration helps maintain fluid dynamics within the body. When well-hydrated, the lymphatic fluid remains more liquid and flows smoothly through the vessels, reducing the risk of stagnation and congestion that can contribute to lymphedema.

3. Preventing Dehydration-Related Complications:

- Dehydration can exacerbate lymphedema symptoms by causing the lymphatic fluid to become thicker and more difficult to transport. This can lead to increased swelling, discomfort, and potential complications such as cellulitis or infections. Proper hydration serves as a preventive measure against these issues.

4. Optimizing Tissue Health:

- Hydration is essential for maintaining the health and elasticity of tissues, including the skin. Well-hydrated tissues are more resilient and less prone to damage, reducing the risk of skin-related complications commonly associated with lymphedema.

5. Supporting Nutrient Transport:

- The lymphatic system plays a crucial role in transporting nutrients and waste products throughout the body. Adequate hydration ensures the efficient transport of essential nutrients to cells and facilitates the removal of waste products, contributing to overall cellular health.

6. Hydration and Exercise:

- Regular, gentle exercise is often recommended for individuals with lymphedema. Hydration supports exercise by maintaining joint lubrication, regulating body temperature, and facilitating the elimination of metabolic byproducts. Combining proper hydration with appropriate exercise can enhance lymphatic function.

7. Maintaining Electrolyte Balance:

- Electrolytes, such as sodium, potassium, and magnesium, play a role in fluid balance within cells and tissues. Proper hydration helps maintain electrolyte balance, reducing the risk of fluid retention and supporting the body's ability to regulate osmotic pressure.

8. Individualized Hydration Goals:

- Hydration needs can vary among individuals, and personalized hydration goals should be established based on factors such as age, weight, activity level, and climate. A healthcare professional or registered dietitian can assist in determining an appropriate and achievable hydration plan for individuals with lymphedema.

9. Strategies for Hydration:

- Individuals with lymphedema should aim for a steady and consistent intake of fluids throughout the day. Water is the primary choice, and beverages with added electrolytes may be beneficial. Monitoring urine color can serve as a simple indicator of hydration status, with pale yellow indicating adequate hydration.

Hydration Tips for Seniors

Seniors must drink enough water since it has a direct impact on many parts of their health, including their physical and mental well-being. Seniors must embrace mindful hydration practices since aging alters the body's water balance and experience of thirst. The following are senior-specific hydration recommendations from professionals:

1. Establish a Regular Hydration Routine:

- Seniors should aim to establish a consistent routine for hydration by incorporating regular water breaks throughout the day. This helps maintain steady fluid intake and prevents dehydration, especially since aging individuals may experience diminished thirst sensation.

2. Monitor Urine Colour:

- Monitoring urine color can serve as a practical indicator of hydration status. Pale yellow urine suggests adequate hydration, while darker urine may indicate the need for increased fluid intake. This simple visual cue can assist seniors in maintaining optimal hydration levels.

3. Incorporate Hydrating Foods:

- Certain fruits and vegetables have high water content and can contribute to overall hydration. Watermelon, cucumbers, oranges, and berries are excellent choices to supplement fluid intake while providing essential nutrients.

4. Choose Beverages Wisely:

- Seniors should prioritize water as their primary beverage. Additionally, incorporating herbal teas, diluted fruit juices, and low-sodium broths can add variety to their fluid intake. Limiting caffeinated and sugary drinks is advisable to avoid potential diuretic effects.

5. Use Hydration Apps or Timers:

- Technology can assist in maintaining hydration goals. Seniors can use hydration reminder apps or set timers on their devices to prompt them to drink water at regular intervals, ensuring consistent fluid intake throughout the day.

6. Consider Electrolyte Balance:

- Maintaining electrolyte balance is crucial, especially for seniors engaging in physical activity. Consuming foods rich in potassium, magnesium, and sodium, alongside proper hydration, can help prevent imbalances and support overall health.

7. Be Mindful of Medication Interactions:

- Certain medications may affect hydration levels or require adjustments in fluid intake. Seniors should consult with healthcare professionals to understand how their medications may impact hydration and receive guidance on maintaining an appropriate balance.

8. **Adapt to Weather Conditions:**

- Environmental factors, such as temperature and humidity, can influence hydration needs. Seniors should be mindful of these conditions and adjust their fluid intake accordingly, especially during hot weather when additional hydration may be necessary.

9. **Use Hydration Aids:**

- For seniors who may face challenges with grip or mobility, using hydration aids such as spill-proof water bottles, straws, or hydration stations strategically placed throughout the living space can facilitate easier access to fluids.

10. **Engage in Social Hydration:**

- Encouraging social activities centered around hydration can be beneficial. Seniors may find it enjoyable to share a cup of tea or water with friends, fostering a supportive environment for maintaining hydration goals.

LIFESTYLE TIPS FOR SENIORS WITH LYMPHEDEMA

Incorporating Gentle Exercise

Keeping an active lifestyle becomes more and more important for general health and vitality as elders age. Modest exercise regimens based on personal requirements and capabilities are essential for maintaining physical health, averting chronic illnesses, and improving overall life satisfaction. Seniors should include modest exercise in their everyday routines, according to standards approved by professionals.

1. **Understanding the Benefits:**

   - Gentle exercise offers a spectrum of benefits for seniors, including improved cardiovascular health, enhanced flexibility, increased muscle strength, and better balance. These benefits contribute to maintaining independence, reducing the risk of falls, and promoting an overall sense of well-being.

2. **Consultation with Healthcare Professionals:**

   - Before initiating any exercise program, seniors should consult with their healthcare professionals. A thorough assessment helps determine the appropriate level of activity, considering individual health conditions, mobility issues, and any specific concerns that may influence the choice of exercise.

3. Choose Low-Impact Activities:

- Low-impact exercises are gentle on the joints and suitable for seniors. Walking, swimming, stationary cycling and tai chi are excellent examples. These activities promote cardiovascular health without placing undue stress on the joints, making them ideal for seniors with arthritis or joint discomfort.

4. Incorporate Strength Training:

- Gentle strength training exercises help maintain muscle mass, bone density, and functional capacity. Resistance bands, light dumbbells, or bodyweight exercises can be incorporated into a routine to improve muscle strength and reduce the risk of frailty.

5. Emphasize Flexibility and Balance:

- Flexibility and balance exercises are crucial for preventing falls and enhancing overall mobility. Stretching routines, yoga, and exercises that focus on balance, such as heel-to-toe walking, contribute to improved flexibility and stability.

6. Mindful Movement Practices:

- Mind-body practices, such as yoga and tai chi, are particularly beneficial for seniors. These exercises not only promote physical well-being but also enhance mental clarity, reduce stress, and foster a sense of relaxation.

7. Adaptations for Mobility Challenges:

- Seniors with mobility challenges can benefit from chair exercises or exercises in the water, which reduce impact and provide additional support. Tailoring exercises to individual needs ensures that everyone, regardless of their mobility level, can engage in physical activity.

8. Establish a Consistent Routine:

- Consistency is key to reaping the benefits of gentle exercise. Seniors should aim for a regular and achievable routine, incorporating activities they enjoy to enhance motivation and adherence to the program.

9. Social Engagement:

- Group exercises or classes offer not only physical benefits but also social engagement, which is essential for mental and emotional well-being. Seniors may find motivation and support in exercising with peers, contributing to a sense of community and shared accomplishment.

10. Monitor Progress and Adapt:

- Regular monitoring of progress allows seniors to adapt their exercise routines based on their evolving needs. Adjustments can be made to accommodate changes in health, mobility, or personal preferences, ensuring that the exercise plan remains safe and effective.

Stress Management and Relaxation Techniques

Stress is a natural part of life, and as people get older, managing stress well becomes increasingly important for preserving general health and quality of life. Stress can worsen pre-existing medical issues and harm the mental health of seniors. To enhance overall feelings of calm and contentment, reduce the harmful effects of stress, and promote resilience, it is imperative to adopt stress management and relaxation strategies.

1. **Understanding the Impact of Stress on Seniors:**

   - Seniors may experience stress due to various factors, including health concerns, lifestyle changes, loss of loved ones, or financial worries. Chronic stress can contribute to conditions such as hypertension, weakened immune function, and exacerbation of existing health issues.

2. **Mindfulness Meditation:**

   - Mindfulness meditation involves cultivating present-moment awareness and acceptance. Seniors can benefit from guided meditation sessions, focusing on breath awareness, body scan techniques, or mindfulness practices tailored to their preferences. Regular practice enhances emotional well-being and reduces stress levels.

3. **Deep Breathing Exercises:**

- Deep breathing exercises, such as diaphragmatic breathing or belly breathing, promote relaxation by activating the body's parasympathetic nervous system. Seniors can practice these techniques regularly to reduce stress, enhance oxygenation, and improve overall respiratory function.

4. **Progressive Muscle Relaxation (PMR):**

- PMR involves systematically tensing and relaxing different muscle groups, promoting physical and mental relaxation. This technique is particularly effective for seniors dealing with muscle tension, anxiety, or insomnia. Regular practice can improve sleep quality and alleviate physical discomfort.

5. **Guided Imagery and Visualization:**

- Seniors can engage in guided imagery or visualization exercises to create mental images that induce relaxation and positive emotions. Imagining peaceful scenes or visualizing the release of stressors can be powerful tools for promoting mental well-being.

6. **Yoga and Tai Chi:**

- Both yoga and tai chi combine gentle movements, breath control, and mindfulness, making them effective stress management tools for seniors. These practices enhance flexibility, balance, and mental focus, contributing to overall physical and emotional well-being.

7. Social Support and Connection:

- Maintaining social connections and seeking support from friends, family, or community groups is vital for stress management. Engaging in activities that foster social bonds provides emotional support, reduces feelings of isolation, and contributes to a sense of belonging.

8. Expressive Arts Therapy:

- Seniors can explore creative outlets such as painting, writing, or music as forms of self-expression and stress relief. Participating in artistic activities can be therapeutic, promoting emotional expression and a sense of accomplishment.

9. Regular Physical Activity:

- Engaging in regular, moderate physical activity is a powerful stress management strategy. Seniors can choose activities such as walking, swimming, or gentle exercise routines to promote the release of endorphins, which act as natural mood enhancers.

10. Cognitive Behavioural Techniques:

- Cognitive-behavioral techniques involve identifying and challenging negative thought patterns. Seniors can work with mental health professionals to develop coping strategies, fostering a more positive and resilient mindset in the face of stressors.

BREAKFAST RECIPES

Quinoa Breakfast Bowl

Ingredients:

- 3/4 cup cooked quinoa
- 1/3 cup diced mango
- 1/5 tablespoons chopped almonds
- 1/1 teaspoons chia seeds
- 1/3 cup low-fat Greek yogurt
- Drizzle of honey (optional)

Cooking Time: 15 minutes

Preparation Time: 7 minutes

Total Time: 22 minutes

Nutritional Information (Per Serving):

- Calories: 450
- Protein: 15g
- Carbohydrates: 67.5g
- Fat: 12g
- Fiber: 9g

Directions:

1. Arrange cooked quinoa in a bowl.

2. Sprinkle chia seeds, sliced almonds, and diced mango on top.

3. Add a generous spoonful of Greek yogurt and, if desired, a touch of honey.

Spinach and Mushroom Omelette

Ingredients:

- 3 eggs

- 3/4 cup fresh spinach, chopped

- 1/3 cup sliced mushrooms

- Salt and pepper to taste

- 1/5 teaspoons Olive oil

Cooking Time: 20 minutes

Preparation Time: 12. minutes

Total Time: 32 minutes

Nutritional Information (Per Serving):

- Calories: 375

- Protein: 27g

- Carbohydrates: 7.5g

- Fat: 27g

- Fiber: 3g

Directions:

1. Whisk the eggs in a bowl, and season with salt and pepper.

2. Heat Olive oil in a nonstick skillet over medium heat.

3. Sauté mushrooms until tender.

4. Add spinach, and cook until wilted.

5. Pour in the whisked eggs, cook until set, and fold the Omelette in half.

Veggie and Cheese Omelette

Ingredients:

- 3 eggs

- 1/3 cup diced bell peppers

- 1/3 cup diced tomatoes

- 1/3 cup diced zucchini

- 1/3 cup shredded low-fat cheese

- 1/5 teaspoons Olive oil

- Salt and pepper to taste

Cooking Time: 15 minutes

Preparation Time: 12 minutes

Total Time: 27 minutes

Nutritional Information (Per Serving):

- Calories: 375

- Protein: 30g

- Fat: 22.5g

- Fiber: 4.5g

Directions:

1. Whisk eggs in a bowl, and season with salt and pepper.

2. Heat Olive oil in a nonstick skillet over medium heat.

3. Sauté diced tomatoes, bell peppers, and zucchini for a few minutes.

4. Pour whisked eggs into the skillet, and sprinkle shredded low-fat cheese on one half.

5. Cover with the other half and cook for an additional minute.

6. Serve hot.

Cottage Cheese and Fruit Bowl

Ingredients:

- 1/5 cup low-fat cottage cheese

- 3/4 cup mixed fruit (pineapple, kiwi, mango)

- 2/5 tablespoons chopped nuts (pecans, cashews)

- 1/5 teaspoons honey

Cooking Time: N/A

Preparation Time: 5 minutes

Total Time: 5 minutes

Nutritional Information (Per Serving):

- Calories: 450

- Protein: 37.5g

- Carbohydrates: 45g

- Fat: 15g

Directions:

1. Spoon low-fat cottage cheese into a bowl.

2. Top with chopped nuts and mixed fruit.

3. Drizzle honey on top.

4. Serve promptly.

Avocado Toast with Poached Egg

Ingredients:

- 1/5 slices whole grain bread, toasted

- 3/4 avocado, mashed

- 1/5 poached eggs

- 1/5 teaspoons olive oil

- Salt and pepper to taste

Cooking Time: 15 minutes

Preparation Time: 12 minutes

Total Time: 27 minutes

Nutritional Information (Per Serving):

- Calories: 450

- Protein: 23.5g

- Carbohydrates: 30g

- Fat: 30g

- Fiber: 9g

Directions:

1. Spread mashed avocado on the toasted bread.

2. Top with poached eggs.

3. Season with salt and pepper, and drizzle with olive oil.

4. Serve promptly.

Vegetable Omelette with Herbs

Ingredients:

- 4 large eggs

- 1 cup mixed vegetables (bell peppers, spinach, tomatoes), finely chopped

- 2 tablespoons chopped fresh herbs (parsley, chives)

- 1 tablespoon olive oil

- Salt and pepper to taste

Prep Time: 15 mins

Total Time: 20 mins

Servings: 2

Nutrition Facts (per serving):

- Calories: 220

- Protein: 14g

- Carbohydrates: 7g

- Fat: 15g

- Fiber: 3g

Directions:

1. Whisk eggs in a bowl and season with salt and pepper.

2. Heat olive oil in a skillet over medium heat.

3. Sauté mixed vegetables until tender.

4. Pour whisked eggs over vegetables and sprinkle with fresh herbs.

5. Cook until eggs are set, then fold the omelet in half.

6. Serve hot.

Chia Seed Pudding with Tropical Fruits

Ingredients:

- 2 tablespoons chia seeds

- 1/2 cup almond milk

- 1/2 cup mixed tropical fruits (pineapple, mango, kiwi)

- 1 tablespoon shredded coconut

Prep Time: 10 mins (plus overnight chilling)

Total Time: 10 mins

Servings: 1

Nutrition Facts (per serving):

- Calories: 280

- Protein: 7g

- Carbohydrates: 35g

- Fat: 14g

- Fiber: 12g

Directions:

1. Mix chia seeds with almond milk in a jar; refrigerate overnight.

2. In the morning, layer chia pudding with mixed tropical fruits.

3. Sprinkle shredded coconut on top.

4. Serve chilled.

Spinach and Feta Breakfast Wrap

Ingredients:

- 1 whole-grain tortilla

- 2 large eggs, scrambled

- 1/2 cup fresh spinach

- 2 tablespoons crumbled feta cheese

- 1 teaspoon olive oil

- Salt and pepper to taste

Prep Time: 12 mins

Total Time: 17 mins

Servings: 1

Nutrition Facts (per serving):

- Calories: 320

- Protein: 18g

- Carbohydrates: 25g

- Fat: 15g

- Fiber: 5g

Directions:

1. Sauté fresh spinach in olive oil until wilted.

2. Scramble eggs and season with salt and pepper.

3. Warm tortilla and layer with scrambled eggs, sautéed spinach, and feta cheese.

4. Roll into a wrap.

5. Serve warm.

Berry Yogurt Parfait

Ingredients:

- 1 cup low-fat Greek yogurt

- 1/2 cup mixed berries (strawberries, blueberries, raspberries)

- 2 tablespoons granola

- 1 tablespoon honey

Prep Time: 12 mins

Total Time: 17 mins

Servings: 1

Nutrition Facts (per serving):

- Calories: 280

- Protein: 18g

- Carbohydrates: 40g

- Fat: 7g

- Fiber: 6g

Directions:

1. Layer Greek yogurt in a glass or bowl.

2. Add mixed berries on top.

3. Sprinkle granola over the berries.

4. Drizzle honey for sweetness.

5. Repeat layers if desired.

6. Serve chilled.

Quinoa and Vegetable Breakfast Bowl

Ingredients:

- 1 cup cooked quinoa

- 1 cup mixed vegetables (broccoli, bell peppers, cherry tomatoes)

- 2 poached eggs

- 1 tablespoon olive oil

- Salt and pepper to taste

Prep Time: 15 mins

Total Time: 25 mins

Servings: 2

Nutrition Facts (per serving):

- Calories: 320

- Protein: 15g

- Carbohydrates: 35g

- Fat: 15g

- Fiber: 7g

Directions:

1. Sauté mixed vegetables in olive oil until tender.

2. Spoon cooked quinoa into bowls.

3. Top with sautéed vegetables and poached eggs.

4. Season with salt and pepper.

5. Serve warm.

LUNCH RECIPES

Quinoa and Chickpea Salad

Ingredients:

- 1 cup cooked quinoa

- 1 can (15 oz) chickpeas, drained and rinsed

- 1 cup cherry tomatoes, halved

- 1 cucumber, diced

- 1/4 cup red onion, finely chopped

- 2 tablespoons olive oil

- 2 tablespoons balsamic vinegar

- Salt and pepper to taste

- Fresh herbs (parsley or mint) for garnish

Prep Time: 15 mins

Cooking Time: 0 mins

Total Time: 15 mins

Servings: 2

Nutrition Facts (per serving):

- Calories: 350

- Protein: 10g

- Carbohydrates: 52g

- Fat: 12g

- Fiber: 10g

Directions:

1. In a large bowl, combine cooked quinoa, chickpeas, cherry tomatoes, cucumber, and red onion.

2. In a small bowl, whisk together olive oil, balsamic vinegar, salt, and pepper.

3. Pour the dressing over the salad and toss until well combined.

4. Garnish with fresh herbs.

5. Serve chilled.

Salmon and Asparagus Foil Packets

Ingredients:

- 2 salmon fillets

- 1 bunch asparagus, trimmed

- 2 tablespoons olive oil

- 2 cloves garlic, minced

- Lemon slices for garnish

- Salt and pepper to taste

- Fresh dill for garnish

Prep Time: 10 mins

Cooking Time: 20 mins

Total Time: 30 mins

Servings: 2

Nutrition Facts (per serving):

- Calories: 400

- Protein: 25g

- Carbohydrates: 8g

- Fat: 30g

- Fiber: 4g

Directions:

1. Preheat oven to 400°F (200°C).

2. Place each salmon fillet on a piece of foil.

3. Arrange asparagus around the salmon.

4. Drizzle olive oil and sprinkle minced garlic over the salmon and asparagus.

5. Season with salt and pepper.

6. Fold the foil to create packets.

7. Bake for 20 minutes or until salmon is cooked through.

8. Garnish with lemon slices and fresh dill.

9. Serve hot.

Mushroom and Spinach Stuffed Chicken Breast

Ingredients:

- 2 boneless, skinless chicken breasts

- 1 cup mushrooms, chopped

- 2 cups fresh spinach

- 1/4 cup feta cheese, crumbled

- 2 tablespoons olive oil

- 2 cloves garlic, minced

- Salt and pepper to taste

- Paprika for seasoning

Prep Time: 20 mins

Cooking Time: 25 mins

Total Time: 45 mins

Servings: 2

Nutrition Facts (per serving):

- Calories: 380

- Protein: 35g

- Carbohydrates: 8g

- Fat: 24g

- Fiber: 3g

Directions:

1. Preheat oven to 375°F (190°C).

2. Butterfly each chicken breast and season with salt, pepper, and paprika.

3. Sauté mushrooms and garlic in olive oil until softened.

4. Add fresh spinach and cook until wilted.

5. Spoon the mushroom and spinach mixture onto each chicken breast.

6. Sprinkle crumbled feta on top.

7. Fold the chicken breasts and secure them with toothpicks.

8. Bake for 25 minutes or until chicken is cooked through.

9. Serve hot.

Vegetarian Lentil Soup

Ingredients:

- 1 cup dry green lentils, rinsed

- 1 onion, diced

- 2 carrots, diced

- 2 celery stalks, diced

- 3 cloves garlic, minced

- 1 can (14 oz) diced tomatoes

- 6 cups vegetable broth

- 1 teaspoon ground cumin

- 1 teaspoon smoked paprika

- Salt and pepper to taste

- Fresh parsley for garnish

Prep Time: 15 mins

Cooking Time: 30 mins

Total Time: 45 mins

Servings: 4

Nutrition Facts (per serving):

- Calories: 300

- Protein: 18g

- Carbohydrates: 52g

- Fat: 2g

- Fiber: 16g

Directions:

1. In a large pot, combine lentils, onion, carrots, celery, garlic, diced tomatoes, vegetable broth, cumin, smoked paprika, salt, and pepper.

2. Bring to a boil, then reduce heat and simmer for 30 minutes or until lentils are tender.

3. Garnish with fresh parsley.

4. Serve hot.

Turkey and Vegetable Stir-Fry

Ingredients:

- 1 lb ground turkey

- 2 cups broccoli florets

- 1 red bell pepper, sliced

- 1 yellow bell pepper, sliced

- 1 cup snap peas

- 3 tablespoons soy sauce

- 2 tablespoons hoisin sauce

- 1 tablespoon sesame oil

- 2 teaspoons grated ginger

- 2 teaspoons minced garlic

- 2 green onions, sliced

- Sesame seeds for garnish

Prep Time: 20 mins

Cooking Time: 15 mins

Total Time: 35 mins

Servings: 4

Nutrition Facts (per serving):

- Calories: 320

- Protein: 25g

- Carbohydrates: 15g

- Fat: 18g

- Fiber: 5g

Directions:

1. In a wok or skillet, brown ground turkey until cooked through.

2. Add broccoli, bell peppers, and snap peas; stir-fry until vegetables are tender-crisp.

3. In a small bowl, mix soy sauce, hoisin sauce, sesame oil, ginger, and garlic.

4. Pour the sauce over the turkey and vegetables; stir to combine.

5. Garnish with sliced green onions and sesame seeds.

6. Serve hot over brown rice or quinoa.

Mediterranean Chickpea Salad

Ingredients:

- 2 cans (15 oz each) chickpeas, drained and rinsed
- 1 cucumber, diced
- 1 cup cherry tomatoes, halved
- 1/2 red onion, finely chopped
- 1/2 cup Kalamata olives, sliced
- 1/2 cup crumbled feta cheese
- 1/4 cup extra virgin olive oil
- 2 tablespoons red wine vinegar
- 1 teaspoon dried oregano
- Salt and pepper to taste
- Fresh parsley for garnish

Prep Time: 15 mins

Cooking Time: 0 mins

Total Time: 15 mins

Servings: 4

Nutrition Facts (per serving):

- Calories: 380
- Protein: 15g

- Carbohydrates: 45g

- Fat: 18g

- Fiber: 12g

Directions:

1. In a large bowl, combine chickpeas, cucumber, cherry tomatoes, red onion, olives, and feta.

2. In a small bowl, whisk together olive oil, red wine vinegar, oregano, salt, and pepper.

3. Pour the dressing over the salad and toss until well combined.

4. Garnish with fresh parsley.

5. Serve chilled.

Grilled Lemon Herb Chicken

Ingredients:

- 2 boneless, skinless chicken breasts

- 2 tablespoons olive oil

- 2 tablespoons lemon juice

- 1 teaspoon dried thyme

- 1 teaspoon dried rosemary

- 1 teaspoon garlic powder

- Salt and pepper to taste

- Lemon wedges for garnish

- Fresh thyme for garnish

Prep Time: 15 mins

Cooking Time: 15 mins

Total Time: 30 mins

Servings: 2

Nutrition Facts (per serving):

- Calories: 320

- Protein: 30g

- Carbohydrates: 2g

- Fat: 21g

- Fiber: 1g

Directions:

1. In a bowl, mix olive oil, lemon juice, thyme, rosemary, garlic powder, salt, and pepper.

2. Marinate chicken breasts in the mixture for at least 15 minutes.

3. Preheat the grill or grill pan over medium-high heat.

4. Grill chicken for about 6-8 minutes per side or until cooked through.

5. Garnish with lemon wedges and fresh thyme.

6. Serve hot.

Shrimp and Quinoa Stir-Fry

Ingredients:

- 1 lb large shrimp, peeled and deveined
- 1 cup cooked quinoa
- 1 cup broccoli florets
- 1 bell pepper, thinly sliced
- 1 carrot, julienned
- 2 tablespoons soy sauce
- 1 tablespoon oyster sauce
- 1 tablespoon sesame oil
- 1 teaspoon grated ginger
- 1 teaspoon minced garlic
- Green onions for garnish
- Sesame seeds for garnish

Prep Time: 20 mins

Cooking Time: 10 mins

Total Time: 30 mins

Servings: 4

Nutrition Facts (per serving):

- Calories: 340

- Protein: 28g

- Carbohydrates: 30g

- Fat: 12g

- Fiber: 5g

Directions:

1. In a wok or skillet, stir-fry shrimp until pink and opaque; set aside.

2. In the same wok, stir-fry broccoli, bell pepper, and carrot until crisp-tender.

3. Add cooked quinoa and soy sauce to the vegetables; stir to combine.

4. Return shrimp to the wok, add oyster sauce, sesame oil, ginger, and garlic; toss until well-coated.

5. Garnish with sliced green onions and sesame seeds.

6. Serve hot.

Tomato Basil Mozzarella Salad

Ingredients:

- 2 cups cherry tomatoes, halved

- 1 cup fresh mozzarella balls

- 1/4 cup fresh basil leaves, torn

- 2 tablespoons balsamic glaze

- 1 tablespoon extra-virgin olive oil

- Salt and pepper to taste

Prep Time: 10 mins

Cooking Time: 0 mins

Total Time: 10 mins

Servings: 2

Nutrition Facts (per serving):

- Calories: 250

- Protein: 14g

- Carbohydrates: 8g

- Fat: 18g

- Fiber: 2g

Directions:

1. In a bowl, combine cherry tomatoes, mozzarella balls, and torn basil leaves.

2. Drizzle with balsamic glaze and olive oil.

3. Season with salt and pepper.

4. Toss gently until well combined.

5. Serve chilled.

Lemon Dill Baked Cod

Ingredients:

- 2 cod fillets

- 2 tablespoons melted butter

- 2 tablespoons lemon juice

- 1 tablespoon fresh dill, chopped

- 1 teaspoon lemon zest

- Salt and pepper to taste

- Lemon wedges for garnish

- Fresh dill for garnish

Prep Time: 10 mins

Cooking Time: 20 mins

Total Time: 30 mins

Servings: 2

Nutrition Facts (per serving):

- Calories: 280

- Protein: 30g

- Carbohydrates: 1g

- Fat: 17g

- Fiber: 0g

Directions:

1. Preheat oven to 400°F (200°C).

2. Place cod fillets on a baking sheet.

3. In a bowl, mix melted butter, lemon juice, chopped dill, lemon zest, salt, and pepper.

4. Brush the cod fillets with the lemon dill mixture.

5. Bake for 15-20 minutes or until the cod is flaky and cooked through.

6. Garnish with lemon wedges and fresh dill.

7. Serve hot.

DINNER RECIPES

Baked Lemon Herb Chicken

Ingredients:

- 4 bone-in, skin-on chicken thighs
- 1 lemon, juiced and zested
- 2 tablespoons olive oil
- 2 teaspoons dried thyme
- 2 teaspoons dried rosemary
- 2 cloves garlic, minced
- Salt and pepper to taste
- Fresh parsley for garnish

Prep Time: 15 mins

Cooking Time: 40 mins

Total Time: 55 mins

Servings: 4

Nutrition Facts (per serving):

- Calories: 380
- Protein: 28g

- Carbohydrates: 2g

- Fat: 30g

- Fiber: 0g

Directions:

1. Preheat oven to 400°F (200°C).

2. In a bowl, mix lemon juice, lemon zest, olive oil, thyme, rosemary, minced garlic, salt, and pepper.

3. Place chicken thighs in a baking dish and pour the lemon herb mixture over them.

4. Bake for 40 minutes or until chicken is golden brown and cooked through.

5. Garnish with fresh parsley.

6. Serve hot.

Vegetarian Stir-Fried Tofu and Broccoli

Ingredients:

- 1 block of firm tofu, pressed and cubed

- 2 cups broccoli florets

- 1 bell pepper, sliced

- 1 carrot, julienned

- 2 tablespoons soy sauce

- 1 tablespoon hoisin sauce

- 1 tablespoon sesame oil

- 1 teaspoon grated ginger

- 1 teaspoon minced garlic

- 2 green onions, sliced

- Sesame seeds for garnish

Prep Time: 25 mins

Cooking Time: 15 mins

Total Time: 40 mins

Servings: 3

Nutrition Facts (per serving):

- Calories: 280

- Protein: 18g

- Carbohydrates: 18g

- Fat: 16g

- Fiber: 6g

Directions:

1. Press tofu to remove excess water, then cut into cubes.

2. In a wok or skillet, stir-fry tofu until golden brown; set aside.

3. Stir-fry broccoli, bell pepper, and carrot until crisp-tender.

4. Add cooked tofu to the vegetables.

5. In a small bowl, mix soy sauce, hoisin sauce, sesame oil, ginger, and garlic; pour over tofu and vegetables.

6. Toss until well-coated.

7. Garnish with sliced green onions and sesame seeds.

8. Serve hot over brown rice or quinoa.

Lentil and Vegetable Curry

Ingredients:

- 1 cup dry green lentils, rinsed

- 1 onion, diced

- 2 carrots, diced

- 2 potatoes, peeled and diced

- 1 can (14 oz) diced tomatoes

- 1 can (14 oz) coconut milk

- 2 tablespoons curry powder

- 1 teaspoon ground turmeric

- 1 teaspoon ground cumin

- Salt and pepper to taste

- Fresh cilantro for garnish

Prep Time: 20 mins

Cooking Time: 30 mins

Total Time: 50 mins

Servings: 4

Nutrition Facts (per serving):

- Calories: 320

- Protein: 14g

- Carbohydrates: 50g

- Fat: 8g

- Fiber: 16g

Directions:

1. In a large pot, combine lentils, onion, carrots, potatoes, diced tomatoes, coconut milk, curry powder, turmeric, cumin, salt, and pepper.

2. Bring to a boil, then reduce heat and simmer for 30 minutes or until lentils are tender.

3. Garnish with fresh cilantro.

4. Serve hot over rice or quinoa.

Baked Turkey Meatballs with Tomato Sauce

Ingredients:

- 1 lb ground turkey

- 1/2 cup breadcrumbs

- 1/4 cup grated Parmesan cheese

- 1 egg, beaten

- 2 cloves garlic, minced

- 1 teaspoon dried oregano

- 1 teaspoon dried basil

- Salt and pepper to taste

- 2 cups tomato sauce

- Fresh basil for garnish

Prep Time: 20 mins

Cooking Time: 25 mins

Total Time: 45 mins

Servings: 4

Nutrition Facts (per serving):

- Calories: 280

- Protein: 22g

- Carbohydrates: 15g

- Fat: 14g

- Fiber: 4g

Directions:

1. Preheat oven to 400°F (200°C).

2. In a bowl, combine ground turkey, breadcrumbs, Parmesan cheese, beaten egg, minced garlic, oregano, basil, salt, and pepper.

3. Shape the mixture into meatballs and place them in a baking dish.

4. Bake for 25 minutes or until meatballs are cooked through.

5. Heat tomato sauce in a saucepan.

6. Pour the sauce over the baked meatballs.

7. Garnish with fresh basil.

8. Serve hot over whole wheat pasta or zucchini noodles.

Grilled Salmon with Lemon Dill Sauce

Ingredients:

- 2 salmon fillets

- 2 tablespoons olive oil

- 2 tablespoons lemon juice

- 1 tablespoon fresh dill, chopped

- 1 teaspoon Dijon mustard

- Salt and pepper to taste

- Lemon wedges for garnish

- Fresh dill for garnish

Prep Time: 15 mins

Cooking Time: 12 mins

Total Time: 27 mins

Servings: 2

Nutrition Facts (per serving):

- Calories: 350

- Protein: 30g

- Carbohydrates: 2g

- Fat: 24g

- Fiber: 0g

Directions:

1. Preheat the grill to medium-high heat.

2. In a bowl, mix olive oil, lemon juice, chopped dill, Dijon mustard, salt, and pepper.

3. Brush salmon fillets with the lemon dill mixture.

4. Grill salmon for about 6 minutes per side or until cooked through.

5. Garnish with lemon wedges and fresh dill.

6. Serve hot.

Quinoa Stuffed Bell Peppers

Ingredients:

- 4 bell peppers, halved and seeds removed
- 1 cup cooked quinoa
- 1 can (15 oz) black beans, drained and rinsed
- 1 cup corn kernels (fresh or frozen)
- 1 cup diced tomatoes
- 1/2 cup shredded cheddar cheese
- 1 teaspoon ground cumin
- 1 teaspoon chili powder
- Salt and pepper to taste
- Fresh cilantro for garnish
- Lime wedges for serving

Prep Time: 20 mins

Cooking Time: 25 mins

Total Time: 45 mins

Servings: 4

Nutrition Facts (per serving):

- Calories: 320
- Protein: 15g

- Carbohydrates: 50g

- Fat: 8g

- Fiber: 12g

Directions:

1. Preheat oven to 375°F (190°C).

2. In a bowl, combine cooked quinoa, black beans, corn, diced tomatoes, shredded cheddar cheese, ground cumin, chili powder, salt, and pepper.

3. Stuff each bell pepper half with the quinoa mixture.

4. Place stuffed peppers in a baking dish.

5. Bake for 25 minutes or until peppers are tender.

6. Garnish with fresh cilantro.

7. Serve hot with lime wedges.

Salmon and Vegetable Foil Packets

Ingredients:

- 2 salmon fillets

- 1 zucchini, sliced

- 1 yellow squash, sliced

- 1 bell pepper, sliced

- 1/2 red onion, sliced

- 2 tablespoons olive oil

- 2 cloves garlic, minced

- 1 teaspoon dried thyme

- Salt and pepper to taste

- Lemon slices for garnish

- Fresh parsley for garnish

Prep Time: 15 mins

Cooking Time: 20 mins

Total Time: 35 mins

Servings: 2

Nutrition Facts (per serving):

- Calories: 350

- Protein: 25g

- Carbohydrates: 15g

- Fat: 20g

- Fiber: 5g

Directions:

1. Preheat oven to 400°F (200°C).

2. Place each salmon fillet on a piece of foil.

3. Arrange zucchini, yellow squash, bell pepper, and red onion around the salmon.

4. Drizzle olive oil and sprinkle minced garlic and dried thyme over the salmon and vegetables.

5. Season with salt and pepper.

6. Fold the foil to create packets.

7. Bake for 20 minutes or until salmon is cooked through.

8. Garnish with lemon slices and fresh parsley.

9. Serve hot.

Vegetable and Quinoa Stuffed Mushrooms

Ingredients:

- 8 large mushrooms, stems removed

- 1 cup cooked quinoa

- 1/2 cup diced bell peppers

- 1/2 cup cherry tomatoes, diced

- 1/4 cup red onion, finely chopped

- 1/4 cup feta cheese, crumbled

- 2 tablespoons olive oil

- 1 teaspoon balsamic vinegar

- 1 teaspoon dried oregano

- Salt and pepper to taste

- Fresh basil for garnish

Prep Time: 20 mins

Cooking Time: 15 mins

Total Time: 35 mins

Servings: 4

Nutrition Facts (per serving):

- Calories: 220

- Protein: 8g

- Carbohydrates: 25g

- Fat: 11g

- Fiber: 4g

Directions:

1. Preheat oven to 375°F (190°C).

2. In a bowl, combine cooked quinoa, diced bell peppers, cherry tomatoes, red onion, feta cheese, olive oil, balsamic vinegar, dried oregano, salt, and pepper.

3. Stuff each mushroom cap with the quinoa mixture.

4. Place stuffed mushrooms in a baking dish.

5. Bake for 15 minutes or until mushrooms are tender.

6. Garnish with fresh basil.

7. Serve hot.

Chicken and Vegetable Skewers

Ingredients:

- 2 boneless, skinless chicken breasts, cut into chunks
- 1 zucchini, sliced
- 1 yellow squash, sliced
- 1 bell pepper, cut into chunks
- 1 red onion, cut into chunks
- 2 tablespoons olive oil
- 1 teaspoon dried Italian herb
- 1 teaspoon garlic powder
- Salt and pepper to taste
- Lemon wedges for serving
- Fresh parsley for garnish

Prep Time: 20 mins

Cooking Time: 15 mins

Total Time: 35 mins

Servings: 4

Nutrition Facts (per serving):

- Calories: 280
- Protein: 28g

- Carbohydrates: 15g

- Fat: 12g

- Fiber: 4g

Directions:

1. Preheat the grill or grill pan over medium-high heat.

2. In a bowl, mix chicken chunks, zucchini, yellow squash, bell pepper, red onion, olive oil, dried Italian herbs, garlic powder, salt, and pepper.

3. Thread the mixture onto skewers.

4. Grill skewers for about 6-8 minutes per side or until chicken is cooked through.

5. Serve with lemon wedges and garnish with fresh parsley.

6. Serve hot.

Turkey and Vegetable Stir-Fry

Ingredients:

- 1 lb ground turkey

- 2 cups broccoli florets

- 1 bell pepper, sliced

- 1 cup snap peas

- 1 carrot, julienned

- 2 tablespoons soy sauce

- 1 tablespoon hoisin sauce

- 1 tablespoon sesame oil

- 1 teaspoon grated ginger

- 1 teaspoon minced garlic

- 2 green onions, sliced

- Sesame seeds for garnish

Prep Time: 20 mins

Cooking Time: 15 mins

Total Time: 35 mins

Servings: 4

Nutrition Facts (per serving):

- Calories: 290

- Protein: 22g

- Carbohydrates: 20g

- Fat: 15g

- Fiber: 5g

Directions:

1. In a wok or skillet, brown ground turkey until cooked through.

2. Add broccoli, bell peppers, snap peas, and carrot; stir-fry until vegetables are tender-crisp.

3. In a small bowl, mix soy sauce, hoisin sauce, sesame oil, ginger, and garlic.

4. Pour the sauce over the turkey and vegetables; stir to combine.

5. Garnish with sliced green onions and sesame seeds.

6. Serve hot over brown rice or quinoa.

Quinoa Stuffed Bell Peppers

Ingredients:

- 4 bell peppers, halved and seeds removed

- 1 cup cooked quinoa

- 1 can (15 oz) black beans, drained and rinsed

- 1 cup corn kernels (fresh or frozen)

- 1 cup diced tomatoes

- 1/2 cup shredded cheddar cheese

- 1 teaspoon ground cumin

- 1 teaspoon chili powder

- Salt and pepper to taste

- Fresh cilantro for garnish

- Lime wedges for serving

Prep Time: 20 mins

Cooking Time: 25 mins

Total Time: 45 mins

Servings: 4

Nutrition Facts (per serving):

- Calories: 320

- Protein: 15g

- Carbohydrates: 50g

- Fat: 8g

- Fiber: 12g

Directions:

1. Preheat oven to 375°F (190°C).

2. In a bowl, combine cooked quinoa, black beans, corn, diced tomatoes, shredded cheddar cheese, ground cumin, chili powder, salt, and pepper.

3. Stuff each bell pepper half with the quinoa mixture.

4. Place stuffed peppers in a baking dish.

5. Bake for 25 minutes or until peppers are tender.

6. Garnish with fresh cilantro.

7. Serve hot with lime wedges.

Salmon and Vegetable Foil Packets

Ingredients:

- 2 salmon fillets

- 1 zucchini, sliced

- 1 yellow squash, sliced

- 1 bell pepper, sliced

- 1/2 red onion, sliced

- 2 tablespoons olive oil

- 2 cloves garlic, minced

- 1 teaspoon dried thyme

- Salt and pepper to taste

- Lemon slices for garnish

- Fresh parsley for garnish

Prep Time: 15 mins

Cooking Time: 20 mins

Total Time: 35 mins

Servings: 2

Nutrition Facts (per serving):

- Calories: 350

- Protein: 25g

- Carbohydrates: 15g

- Fat: 20g

- Fiber: 5g

Directions:

1. Preheat oven to 400°F (200°C).

2. Place each salmon fillet on a piece of foil.

3. Arrange zucchini, yellow squash, bell pepper, and red onion around the salmon.

4. Drizzle olive oil and sprinkle minced garlic and dried thyme over the salmon and vegetables.

5. Season with salt and pepper.

6. Fold the foil to create packets.

7. Bake for 20 minutes or until salmon is cooked through.

8. Garnish with lemon slices and fresh parsley.

9. Serve hot.

Vegetable and Quinoa Stuffed Mushrooms

Ingredients:

- 8 large mushrooms, stems removed

- 1 cup cooked quinoa

- 1/2 cup diced bell peppers

- 1/2 cup cherry tomatoes, diced

- 1/4 cup red onion, finely chopped

- 1/4 cup feta cheese, crumbled

- 2 tablespoons olive oil

- 1 teaspoon balsamic vinegar

- 1 teaspoon dried oregano

- Salt and pepper to taste

- Fresh basil for garnish

Prep Time: 20 mins

Cooking Time: 15 mins

Total Time: 35 mins

Servings: 4

Nutrition Facts (per serving):

- Calories: 220

- Protein: 8g

- Carbohydrates: 25g

- Fat: 11g

- Fiber: 4g

Directions:

1. Preheat oven to 375°F (190°C).

2. In a bowl, combine cooked quinoa, diced bell peppers, cherry tomatoes, red onion, feta cheese, olive oil, balsamic vinegar, dried oregano, salt, and pepper.

3. Stuff each mushroom cap with the quinoa mixture.

4. Place stuffed mushrooms in a baking dish.

5. Bake for 15 minutes or until mushrooms are tender.

6. Garnish with fresh basil.

7. Serve hot.

Chicken and Vegetable Skewers

Ingredients:

- 2 boneless, skinless chicken breasts, cut into chunks

- 1 zucchini, sliced

- 1 yellow squash, sliced

- 1 bell pepper, cut into chunks

- 1 red onion, cut into chunks

- 2 tablespoons olive oil

- 1 teaspoon dried Italian herb

- 1 teaspoon garlic powder

- Salt and pepper to taste

- Lemon wedges for serving

- Fresh parsley for garnish

Prep Time: 20 mins

Cooking Time: 15 mins

Total Time: 35 mins

Servings: 4

Nutrition Facts (per serving):

- Calories: 280

- Protein: 28g

- Carbohydrates: 15g

- Fat: 12g

- Fiber: 4g

Directions:

1. Preheat the grill or grill pan over medium-high heat.

2. In a bowl, mix chicken chunks, zucchini, yellow squash, bell pepper, red onion, olive oil, dried Italian herbs, garlic powder, salt, and pepper.

3. Thread the mixture onto skewers.

4. Grill skewers for about 6-8 minutes per side or until chicken is cooked through.

5. Serve with lemon wedges and garnish with fresh parsley.

6. Serve hot.

Turkey and Vegetable Stir-Fry

Ingredients:

- 1 lb ground turkey

- 2 cups broccoli florets

- 1 bell pepper, sliced

- 1 cup snap peas

- 1 carrot, julienned

- 2 tablespoons soy sauce

- 1 tablespoon hoisin sauce

- 1 tablespoon sesame oil

- 1 teaspoon grated ginger

- 1 teaspoon minced garlic

- 2 green onions, sliced

- Sesame seeds for garnish

Prep Time: 20 mins

Cooking Time: 15 mins

Total Time: 35 mins

Servings: 4

Nutrition Facts (per serving):

- Calories: 290

- Protein: 22g

- Carbohydrates: 20g

- Fat: 15g

- Fiber: 5g

Directions:

1. In a wok or skillet, brown ground turkey until cooked through.

2. Add broccoli, bell peppers, snap peas, and carrot; stir-fry until vegetables are tender-crisp.

3. In a small bowl, mix soy sauce, hoisin sauce, sesame oil, ginger, and garlic.

4. Pour the sauce over the turkey and vegetables; stir to combine.

5. Garnish with sliced green onions and sesame seeds.

6. Serve hot over brown rice or quinoa.

DESSERT RECIPES

Chia Seed Pudding with Mixed Berries

Ingredients:

- 1/4 cup chia seeds

- 1 cup almond milk

- 1 teaspoon vanilla extract

- 1 tablespoon maple syrup

- 1/2 cup mixed berries (strawberries, blueberries, raspberries)

- 1 tablespoon sliced almonds (optional)

- Fresh mint leaves for garnish

Prep Time: 10 mins

Total Time: 4 hours (including chilling time)

Servings: 2

Nutrition Facts (per serving):

- Calories: 180

- Protein: 4g

- Carbohydrates: 20g

- Fat: 9g

- Fiber: 10g

Directions:

1. In a bowl, mix chia seeds, almond milk, vanilla extract, and maple syrup.

2. Stir well and let it sit for 5 minutes, then stir again to prevent clumping.

3. Cover and refrigerate for at least 4 hours or overnight.

4. Before serving, stir the pudding and divide it into serving bowls.

5. Top with mixed berries, sliced almonds (if desired), and fresh mint leaves.

6. Serve chilled.

Baked Apple with Cinnamon and Walnuts

Ingredients:

- 2 apples, cored and halved

- 1 tablespoon melted coconut oil

- 1 teaspoon ground cinnamon

- 2 tablespoons chopped walnuts

- 1 tablespoon honey (optional)

- Greek yogurt for serving

Prep Time: 10 mins

Cooking Time: 25 mins

Total Time: 35 mins

Servings: 2

Nutrition Facts (per serving):

- Calories: 200

- Protein: 2g

- Carbohydrates: 25g

- Fat: 12g

- Fiber: 5g

Directions:

1. Preheat oven to 375°F (190°C).

2. Place apple halves on a baking sheet.

3. Brush melted coconut oil over the apples.

4. Sprinkle ground cinnamon and chopped walnuts over the apples.

5. Bake for 25 minutes or until apples are tender.

6. Drizzle honey on top (if desired).

7. Serve warm with a dollop of Greek yogurt.

Dark Chocolate Avocado Mousse

Ingredients:

- 2 ripe avocados

- 1/4 cup unsweetened cocoa powder

- 1/4 cup maple syrup

- 1 teaspoon vanilla extract

- 1/4 cup almond milk

- Pinch of salt

- Fresh berries for garnish

Prep Time: 10 mins

Total Time: 10 mins

Servings: 4

Nutrition Facts (per serving):

- Calories: 180

- Protein: 3g

- Carbohydrates: 20g

- Fat: 12g

- Fiber: 7g

Directions:

1. In a blender, combine avocados, cocoa powder, maple syrup, vanilla extract, almond milk, and a pinch of salt.

2. Blend until smooth and creamy.

3. Divide the mousse into serving cups.

4. Refrigerate for at least 1 hour to chill.

5. Garnish with fresh berries before serving.

6. Serve chilled.

Oatmeal Raisin Cookies

Ingredients:

- 1 cup old-fashioned oats

- 1/2 cup whole wheat flour

- 1/2 teaspoon baking soda

- 1/2 teaspoon ground cinnamon

- Pinch of salt

- 1/4 cup coconut oil, melted

- 1/4 cup maple syrup

- 1 egg

- 1 teaspoon vanilla extract

- 1/2 cup raisins

Prep Time: 15 mins

Cooking Time: 10 mins

Total Time: 25 mins

Servings: 12

Nutrition Facts (per serving):

- Calories: 120

- Protein: 2g

- Carbohydrates: 18g

- Fat: 5g

- Fiber: 2g

Directions:

1. Preheat oven to 350°F (180°C).

2. In a bowl, combine oats, whole wheat flour, baking soda, ground cinnamon, and a pinch of salt.

3. In another bowl, mix melted coconut oil, maple syrup, egg, and vanilla extract.

4. Add the wet ingredients to the dry ingredients and stir until well combined.

5. Fold in raisins.

6. Drop a spoonful of dough onto a lined baking sheet.

7. Bake for 10 minutes or until golden brown.

8. Allow cookies to cool before serving.

Baked Pear with Honey and Walnuts

Ingredients:

- 2 ripe pears, halved and cored

- 2 tablespoons melted coconut oil

- 2 tablespoons honey

- 1/4 cup chopped walnuts

- Greek yogurt for serving

Prep Time: 10 mins

Cooking Time: 20 mins

Total Time: 30 mins

Servings: 2

Nutrition Facts (per serving):

- Calories: 220

- Protein: 3g

- Carbohydrates: 30g

- Fat: 12g

- Fiber: 6g

Directions:

1. Preheat oven to 375°F (190°C).

2. Place pear halves on a baking sheet.

3. Brush melted coconut oil over the pears.

4. Drizzle honey and sprinkle chopped walnuts over the pears.

5. Bake for 20 minutes or until pears are tender.

6. Serve warm with a dollop of Greek yogurt.

Coconut Chia Seed Popsicles

Ingredients:

- 1/4 cup chia seeds

- 1 can (14 oz) coconut milk

- 2 tablespoons honey

- 1/2 teaspoon vanilla extract

- 1/2 cup mixed tropical fruits (pineapple, mango, kiwi)

- Popsicle molds and sticks

Prep Time: 10 mins

Total Time: 6 hours (including freezing time)

Servings: 4

Nutrition Facts (per serving):

- Calories: 180

- Protein: 3g

- Carbohydrates: 15g

- Fat: 12g

- Fiber: 6g

Directions:

1. In a bowl, mix chia seeds, coconut milk, honey, and vanilla extract.

2. Stir well and let it sit for 5 minutes, then stir again to prevent clumping.

3. Cover and refrigerate for at least 6 hours or overnight.

4. Before filling the molds, stir the mixture once more.

5. Spoon mixed tropical fruits into the bottom of each popsicle mold.

6. Pour the chia seed mixture over the fruits.

7. Insert popsicle sticks and freeze for at least 4 hours.

8. Run molds under warm water to release the popsicles.

9. Serve frozen.

Almond Flour Banana Muffins

Ingredients:

- 2 cups almond flour

- 1 teaspoon baking powder

- 1/2 teaspoon baking soda

- 1/4 teaspoon salt

- 3 ripe bananas, mashed

- 1/4 cup coconut oil, melted

- 1/4 cup maple syrup

- 2 large eggs

- 1 teaspoon vanilla extract

- 1/2 cup chopped walnuts (optional)

Prep Time: 15 mins

Baking Time: 20 mins

Total Time: 35 mins

Servings: 12

Nutrition Facts (per serving):

- Calories: 180

- Protein: 5g

- Carbohydrates: 14g

- Fat: 12g

- Fiber: 3g

Directions:

1. Preheat oven to 350°F (180°C). Line a muffin tin with paper liners.

2. In a bowl, whisk together almond flour, baking powder, baking soda, and salt.

3. In another bowl, mix mashed bananas, melted coconut oil, maple syrup, eggs, and vanilla extract.

4. Add the wet ingredients to the dry ingredients and stir until just combined.

5. Fold in chopped walnuts if desired.

6. Spoon the batter into muffin cups, filling each about 3/4 full.

7. Bake for 20 minutes or until a toothpick inserted comes out clean.

8. Allow muffins to cool before serving.

Berry Parfait with Greek Yogurt

Ingredients:

- 1 cup mixed berries (strawberries, blueberries, raspberries)

- 1 cup low-fat Greek yogurt

- 1/4 cup granola

- 1 tablespoon honey

- Fresh mint leaves for garnish

Prep Time: 10 mins

Total Time: 10 mins

Servings: 2

Nutrition Facts (per serving):

- Calories: 180

- Protein: 15g

- Carbohydrates: 25g

- Fat: 4g

- Fiber: 5g

Directions:

1. In serving glasses or bowls, layer Greek yogurt, mixed berries, and granola.

2. Drizzle honey over each layer.

3. Repeat the layers until the glasses are filled.

4. Garnish with fresh mint leaves.

5. Serve chilled.

Pumpkin Spice Chia Seed Pudding

Ingredients:

- 1/4 cup chia seeds

- 1 cup almond milk

- 1/4 cup canned pumpkin puree

- 2 tablespoons maple syrup

- 1/2 teaspoon pumpkin pie spice

- 1/4 cup chopped pecans

- Whipped coconut cream for topping

Prep Time: 10 mins

Total Time: 4 hours (including chilling time)

Servings: 2

Nutrition Facts (per serving):

- Calories: 220

- Protein: 4g

- Carbohydrates: 20g

- Fat: 14g

- Fiber: 8g

Directions:

1. In a bowl, mix chia seeds, almond milk, pumpkin puree, maple syrup, and pumpkin pie spice.

2. Stir well and let it sit for 5 minutes, then stir again to prevent clumping.

3. Cover and refrigerate for at least 4 hours or overnight.

4. Before serving, stir the pudding and divide it into serving bowls.

5. Top with chopped pecans and a dollop of whipped coconut cream.

6. Serve chilled.

Baked Peach with Cinnamon and Almonds

Ingredients:

- 2 ripe peaches, halved and pitted

- 1 tablespoon melted coconut oil

- 1 teaspoon ground cinnamon

- 2 tablespoons sliced almonds

- 1 tablespoon agave syrup

- Coconut yogurt for serving

Prep Time: 10 mins

Cooking Time: 20 mins

Total Time: 30 mins

Servings: 2

Nutrition Facts (per serving):

- Calories: 190

- Protein: 3g

- Carbohydrates: 25g

- Fat: 10g

- Fiber: 4g

Directions:

1. Preheat oven to 375°F (190°C).

2. Place peach halves on a baking sheet.

3. Brush melted coconut oil over the peaches.

4. Sprinkle ground cinnamon and sliced almonds over the peaches.

5. Drizzle agave syrup on top.

6. Bake for 20 minutes or until peaches are tender.

7. Serve warm with a dollop of coconut yogurt.

SOUP RECIPES

Vegetable Quinoa Soup

Ingredients:

- 1 cup quinoa, rinsed

- 1 tablespoon olive oil

- 1 onion, diced

- 2 carrots, sliced

- 2 celery stalks, chopped

- 2 cloves garlic, minced

- 6 cups low-sodium vegetable broth

- 1 can (14 oz) diced tomatoes

- 1 teaspoon dried thyme

- 1 teaspoon dried oregano

- Salt and pepper to taste

- 2 cups kale, chopped

- 1 can (15 oz) chickpeas, drained and rinsed

Prep Time: 15 mins

Cooking Time: 25 mins

Total Time: 40 mins

Servings: 6

Nutrition Facts (per serving):

- Calories: 280

- Protein: 10g

- Carbohydrates: 45g

- Fat: 7g

- Fiber: 8g

Directions:

1. Rinse quinoa under cold water and set aside.

2. In a large pot, heat olive oil over medium heat. Add onion, carrots, celery, and garlic. Sauté until vegetables are tender.

3. Add vegetable broth, diced tomatoes, dried thyme, dried oregano, salt, and pepper. Bring to a boil.

4. Stir in quinoa, reduce heat, cover, and simmer for 15-20 minutes or until quinoa is cooked.

5. Add kale and chickpeas, and simmer for an additional 5 minutes.

6. Adjust seasoning if needed and serve hot.

Creamy Broccoli and Cauliflower Soup

Ingredients:

- 1 tablespoon olive oil

- 1 onion, diced

- 2 cloves garlic, minced

- 4 cups broccoli florets

- 3 cups cauliflower florets

- 4 cups low-sodium vegetable broth

- 1 cup unsweetened almond milk

- Salt and pepper to taste

- 1/4 cup nutritional yeast (optional, for added flavor)

- Fresh parsley for garnish

Prep Time: 15 mins

Cooking Time: 25 mins

Total Time: 40 mins

Servings: 4

Nutrition Facts (per serving):

- Calories: 180

- Protein: 8g

- Carbohydrates: 20g

- Fat: 9g

- Fiber: 7g

Directions:

1. In a large pot, heat olive oil over medium heat. Add onion and garlic, and sauté until softened.

2. Add broccoli, cauliflower, vegetable broth, almond milk, salt, and pepper. Bring to a boil.

3. Reduce heat, cover, and simmer for 20 minutes or until vegetables are tender.

4. Use an immersion blender to blend the soup until smooth.

5. Stir in nutritional yeast if desired. Adjust seasoning.

6. Garnish with fresh parsley and serve hot.

Lentil and Vegetable Soup

Ingredients:

- 1 cup dried green lentils, rinsed

- 1 tablespoon olive oil

- 1 onion, diced

- 2 carrots, sliced

- 2 celery stalks, chopped

- 2 cloves garlic, minced

- 1 teaspoon ground cumin

- 1 teaspoon smoked paprika

- 6 cups low-sodium vegetable broth

- 1 can (14 oz) diced tomatoes

- Salt and pepper to taste

- 2 cups spinach, chopped

- Fresh lemon wedges for serving

Prep Time: 20 mins

Cooking Time: 30 mins

Total Time: 50 mins

Servings: 6

Nutrition Facts (per serving):

- Calories: 250

- Protein: 14g

- Carbohydrates: 40g

- Fat: 4g

- Fiber: 12g

Directions:

1. In a large pot, heat olive oil over medium heat. Add onion, carrots, celery, and garlic. Sauté until vegetables are softened.

2. Add ground cumin, smoked paprika, lentils, vegetable broth, diced tomatoes, salt, and pepper. Bring to a boil.

3. Reduce heat, cover, and simmer for 25-30 minutes or until lentils are cooked.

4. Stir in chopped spinach and cook for an additional 5 minutes.

5. Adjust seasoning and serve hot with fresh lemon wedges.

Chicken and Rice Soup

Ingredients:

- 1 tablespoon olive oil

- 1 onion, diced

- 2 carrots, sliced

- 2 celery stalks, chopped

- 2 cloves garlic, minced

- 6 cups low-sodium chicken broth

- 1 cup cooked chicken breast, shredded

- 1/2 cup brown rice, cooked

- 1 teaspoon dried thyme

- Salt and pepper to taste

- Fresh parsley for garnish

Prep Time: 20 mins

Cooking Time: 30 mins

Total Time: 50 mins

Servings: 4

Nutrition Facts (per serving):

- Calories: 280

- Protein: 18g

- Carbohydrates: 30g

- Fat: 8g

- Fiber: 5g

Directions:

1. In a large pot, heat olive oil over medium heat. Add onion, carrots, celery, and garlic. Sauté until vegetables are softened.

2. Add chicken broth, shredded chicken, cooked brown rice, dried thyme, salt, and pepper. Bring to a boil.

3. Reduce heat, cover, and simmer for 20 minutes.

4. Adjust seasoning if needed and serve hot with fresh parsley.

Tomato Basil Soup

Ingredients:

- 1 tablespoon olive oil

- 1 onion, diced

- 2 cloves garlic, minced

- 2 cans (28 oz each) of crushed tomatoes

- 4 cups low-sodium vegetable broth

- 1 teaspoon dried basil

- 1/2 teaspoon dried oregano

- Salt and pepper to taste

- 1/4 cup fresh basil, chopped

- Greek yogurt for garnish

Prep Time: 15 mins

Cooking Time: 25 mins

Total Time: 40 mins

Servings: 4

Nutrition Facts (per serving):

- Calories: 150

- Protein: 3g

- Carbohydrates: 25g

- Fat: 5g

- Fiber: 6g

Directions:

1. In a large pot, heat olive oil over medium heat. Add onion and garlic, and sauté until softened.

2. Add crushed tomatoes, vegetable broth, dried basil, dried oregano, salt, and pepper. Bring to a boil.

3. Reduce heat, cover, and simmer for 20 minutes.

4. Use an immersion blender to blend the soup until smooth.

5. Stir in fresh basil and adjust the seasoning.

6. Serve hot, garnished with a dollop of Greek yogurt.

Mushroom and Barley Soup

Ingredients:

- 1 cup pearl barley, rinsed

- 1 tablespoon olive oil

- 1 onion, diced

- 2 carrots, sliced

- 2 celery stalks, chopped

- 8 oz cremini mushrooms, sliced

- 2 cloves garlic, minced

- 6 cups low-sodium vegetable broth

- 1 teaspoon dried thyme

- Salt and pepper to taste

- Fresh parsley for garnish

Prep Time: 15 mins

Cooking Time: 35 mins

Total Time: 50 mins

Servings: 6

Nutrition Facts (per serving):

- Calories: 220

- Protein: 7g

- Carbohydrates: 45g

- Fat: 3g

- Fiber: 10g

Directions:

1. In a large pot, heat olive oil over medium heat. Add onion, carrots, celery, and garlic. Sauté until vegetables are softened.

2. Add sliced mushrooms and cook until they release their moisture.

3. Stir in pearl barley, vegetable broth, dried thyme, salt, and pepper. Bring to a boil.

4. Reduce heat, cover, and simmer for 25-30 minutes or until barley is tender.

5. Adjust seasoning and serve hot, garnished with fresh parsley.

Spinach and Lentil Soup

Ingredients:

- 1 cup dried green lentils, rinsed

- 1 tablespoon olive oil

- 1 onion, diced

- 2 carrots, sliced

- 2 celery stalks, chopped

- 2 cloves garlic, minced

- 6 cups low-sodium vegetable broth

- 4 cups fresh spinach, chopped

- 1 teaspoon ground cumin

- 1/2 teaspoon smoked paprika

- Salt and pepper to taste

- Lemon wedges for serving

Prep Time: 20 mins

Cooking Time: 30 mins

Total Time: 50 mins

Servings: 6

Nutrition Facts (per serving):

- Calories: 250

- Protein: 15g

- Carbohydrates: 40g

- Fat: 4g

- Fiber: 14g

Directions:

1. In a large pot, heat olive oil over medium heat. Add onion, carrots, celery, and garlic. Sauté until vegetables are softened.

2. Add ground cumin, smoked paprika, lentils, vegetable broth, salt, and pepper. Bring to a boil.

3. Reduce heat, cover, and simmer for 25-30 minutes or until lentils are cooked.

4. Stir in chopped spinach and cook until wilted.

5. Adjust seasoning and serve hot with a squeeze of lemon.

Butternut Squash and Apple Soup

Ingredients:

- 1 butternut squash, peeled, seeded, and diced

- 2 apples, peeled, cored, and diced

- 1 onion, diced

- 2 tablespoons olive oil

- 4 cups low-sodium vegetable broth

- 1 teaspoon ground cinnamon

- 1/2 teaspoon nutmeg

- Salt and pepper to taste

- 1/4 cup pumpkin seeds for garnish

Prep Time: 20 mins

Cooking Time: 30 mins

Total Time: 50 mins

Servings: 4

Nutrition Facts (per serving):

- Calories: 180

- Protein: 3g

- Carbohydrates: 35g

- Fat: 6g

- Fiber: 8g

Directions:

1. In a large pot, heat olive oil over medium heat. Add onion and sauté until softened.

2. Add diced butternut squash and apples, and cook for 5 minutes.

3. Pour in vegetable broth, ground cinnamon, nutmeg, salt, and pepper. Bring to a boil.

4. Reduce heat, cover, and simmer for 20-25 minutes or until squash is tender.

5. Use an immersion blender to blend the soup until smooth.

6. Adjust seasoning, garnish with pumpkin seeds, and serve hot.

Creamy Asparagus Soup

Ingredients:

- 1 bunch asparagus, trimmed and chopped

- 1 tablespoon olive oil

- 1 onion, diced

- 2 cloves garlic, minced

- 4 cups low-sodium vegetable broth

- 1 cup unsweetened almond milk

- 2 tablespoons nutritional yeast

- Salt and pepper to taste

- Fresh chives for garnish

Prep Time: 15 mins

Cooking Time: 25 mins

Total Time: 40 mins

Servings: 4

Nutrition Facts (per serving):

- Calories: 160

- Protein: 8g

- Carbohydrates: 20g

- Fat: 7g

- Fiber: 6g

Directions:

1. In a large pot, heat olive oil over medium heat. Add onion and garlic, and sauté until softened.

2. Add chopped asparagus and cook for 5 minutes.

3. Pour in vegetable broth, almond milk, nutritional yeast, salt, and pepper. Bring to a boil.

4. Reduce heat, cover, and simmer for 15-20 minutes or until asparagus is tender.

5. Use an immersion blender to blend the soup until creamy.

6. Adjust seasoning, garnish with fresh chives, and serve hot.

Sweet Potato and Ginger Soup

Ingredients:

- 2 large sweet potatoes, peeled and diced

- 1 tablespoon olive oil

- 1 onion, diced

- 2 cloves garlic, minced

- 1 tablespoon fresh ginger, grated

- 4 cups low-sodium vegetable broth

- 1 can (14 oz) coconut milk

- Salt and pepper to taste

- Fresh cilantro for garnish

Prep Time: 20 mins

Cooking Time: 30 mins

Total Time: 50 mins

Servings: 4

Nutrition Facts (per serving):

- Calories: 220

- Protein: 3g

- Carbohydrates: 35g

- Fat: 8g

- Fiber: 6g

Directions:

1. In a large pot, heat olive oil over medium heat. Add onion, garlic, and ginger. Sauté until softened.

2. Add diced sweet potatoes and cook for 5 minutes.

3. Pour in vegetable broth and coconut milk. Bring to a boil.

4. Reduce heat, cover, and simmer for 20-25 minutes or until sweet potatoes are soft.

5. Use an immersion blender to blend the soup until smooth.

6. Adjust seasoning, garnish with fresh cilantro, and serve hot.

SMOOTHIE RECIPES

Berry Blast Smoothie

Ingredients:

- 1 cup mixed berries (strawberries, blueberries, raspberries)
- 1/2 banana, peeled
- 1/2 cup low-fat Greek yogurt
- 1 tablespoon chia seeds
- 1 cup unsweetened almond milk
- 1 teaspoon honey (optional)
- Ice cubes (optional)

Prep Time: 5 mins

Total Time: 5 mins

Servings: 1

Nutrition Facts (per serving):

- Calories: 180
- Protein: 8g
- Carbohydrates: 30g
- Fat: 4g

- Fiber: 8g

Directions:

1. In a blender, combine mixed berries, bananas, Greek yogurt, chia seeds, almond milk, and honey.

2. Blend until smooth and creamy.

3. Add ice cubes if desired and blend again.

4. Pour into a glass and enjoy this refreshing berry blast.

Green Power Smoothie

Ingredients:

- 1 cup spinach leaves

- 1/2 cucumber, peeled and sliced

- 1/2 green apple, cored and chopped

- 1/2 avocado, peeled and diced

- 1 tablespoon flaxseeds

- 1 cup coconut water

- Juice of 1/2 lemon

- Ice cubes (optional)

Prep Time: 7 mins

Total Time: 7 mins

Servings: 1

Nutrition Facts (per serving):

- Calories: 220

- Protein: 6g

- Carbohydrates: 25g

- Fat: 13g

- Fiber: 9g

Directions:

1. In a blender, combine spinach leaves, cucumber, green apple, avocado, flaxseeds, coconut water, and lemon juice.

2. Blend until smooth and creamy.

3. Add ice cubes if desired and blend again.

4. Pour into a glass and enjoy the nutrient-packed green power smoothie.

Tropical Paradise Smoothie

Ingredients:

- 1/2 cup pineapple chunks

- 1/2 cup mango chunks

- 1/2 banana, peeled

- 1/2 cup coconut milk

- 1 tablespoon shredded coconut

- 1 tablespoon hemp seeds

- Ice cubes (optional)

Prep Time: 6 mins

Total Time: 6 mins

Servings: 1

Nutrition Facts (per serving):

- Calories: 250

- Protein: 7g

- Carbohydrates: 35g

- Fat: 11g

- Fiber: 6g

Directions:

1. In a blender, combine pineapple chunks, mango chunks, banana, coconut milk, shredded coconut, and hemp seeds.

2. Blend until smooth and creamy.

3. Add ice cubes if desired and blend again.

4. Pour into a glass and transport yourself to a tropical paradise with this delicious smoothie.

Creamy Blueberry Almond Smoothie

Ingredients:

- 1 cup blueberries

- 1/4 cup almonds, soaked

- 1/2 cup plain Greek yogurt

- 1 tablespoon almond butter

- 1 cup almond milk

- 1 teaspoon maple syrup (optional)

- Ice cubes (optional)

Prep Time: 8 mins

Total Time: 8 mins

Servings: 1

Nutrition Facts (per serving):

- Calories: 280

- Protein: 14g

- Carbohydrates: 30g

- Fat: 14g

- Fiber: 6g

Directions:

1. In a blender, combine blueberries, soaked almonds, Greek yogurt, almond butter, almond milk, and maple syrup.

2. Blend until smooth and creamy.

3. Add ice cubes if desired and blend again.

4. Pour into a glass and savor the creamy goodness of this blueberry almond smoothie.

Peachy Keen Protein Smoothie

Ingredients:

- 1 cup frozen peaches
- 1/2 cup cottage cheese
- 1/2 cup almond milk
- 1 tablespoon chia seeds
- 1 scoop vanilla protein powder
- 1 teaspoon honey (optional)
- Ice cubes (optional)

Prep Time: 5 mins

Total Time: 5 mins

Servings: 1

Nutrition Facts (per serving):

- Calories: 300
- Protein: 25g
- Carbohydrates: 30g
- Fat: 10g
- Fiber: 7g

Directions:

1. In a blender, combine frozen peaches, cottage cheese, almond milk, chia seeds, protein powder, and honey.

2. Blend until smooth and creamy.

3. Add ice cubes if desired and blend again.

4. Pour into a glass and enjoy this peachy keen protein smoothie for a satisfying and nutritious treat.

Citrus Sunshine Smoothie

Ingredients:

- 1 orange, peeled and segmented

- 1/2 grapefruit, peeled and segmented

- 1/2 cup pineapple chunks

- 1/2 banana, peeled

- 1/2 cup coconut water

- 1 tablespoon flaxseeds

- Ice cubes (optional)

Prep Time: 6 mins

Total Time: 6 mins

Servings: 1

Nutrition Facts (per serving):

- Calories: 200

- Protein: 4g

- Carbohydrates: 40g

- Fat: 3g

- Fiber: 8g

Directions:

1. In a blender, combine orange segments, grapefruit segments, pineapple chunks, banana, coconut water, and flaxseeds.

2. Blend until smooth and refreshing.

3. Add ice cubes if desired and blend again.

4. Pour into a glass and start your day with the sunny flavors of this citrus sunshine smoothie.

Protein-Packed Berry Delight

Ingredients:

- 1 cup mixed berries (strawberries, blueberries, raspberries)

- 1/2 cup cottage cheese

- 1/2 cup almond milk

- 1 scoop vanilla protein powder

- 1 tablespoon almond butter

- 1 teaspoon honey (optional)

- Ice cubes (optional)

Prep Time: 7 mins

Total Time: 7 mins

Servings: 1

Nutrition Facts (per serving):

- Calories: 280

- Protein: 26g

- Carbohydrates: 25g

- Fat: 11g

- Fiber: 6g

Directions:

1. In a blender, combine mixed berries, cottage cheese, almond milk, protein powder, almond butter, and honey.

2. Blend until smooth and packed with protein.

3. Add ice cubes if desired and blend again.

4. Pour into a glass and relish the berry delight.

Minty Green Detox Smoothie

Ingredients:

- 1 cup kale leaves, stems removed

- 1/2 cucumber, peeled and sliced

- 1/2 pear, cored and chopped

- 1/2 lime, juiced

- 1 tablespoon fresh mint leaves

- 1 cup coconut water

- Ice cubes (optional)

Prep Time: 8 mins

Total Time: 8 mins

Servings: 1

Nutrition Facts (per serving):

- Calories: 150

- Protein: 5g

- Carbohydrates: 30g

- Fat: 1g

- Fiber: 7g

Directions:

1. In a blender, combine kale leaves, cucumber, pear, lime juice, mint leaves, and coconut water.

2. Blend until smooth and detoxifying.

3. Add ice cubes if desired and blend again.

4. Pour into a glass and enjoy the refreshing taste of this minty green detox smoothie.

Choco-Banana Bliss Smoothie

Ingredients:

- 1 banana, peeled

- 2 tablespoons cocoa powder

- 1/4 cup rolled oats

- 1 tablespoon almond butter

- 1 cup almond milk

- 1 teaspoon honey (optional)

- Ice cubes (optional)

Prep Time: 6 mins

Total Time: 6 mins

Servings: 1

Nutrition Facts (per serving):

- Calories: 250

- Protein: 7g

- Carbohydrates: 40g

- Fat: 9g

- Fiber: 6g

Directions:

1. In a blender, combine banana, cocoa powder, rolled oats, almond butter, almond milk, and honey.

2. Blend until smooth and indulgent.

3. Add ice cubes if desired and blend again.

4. Pour into a glass and experience the choco-banana bliss.

Pineapple Coconut Paradise Smoothie

Ingredients:

- 1 cup pineapple chunks

- 1/2 cup coconut milk

- 1/4 cup shredded coconut

- 1/2 banana, peeled

- 1 tablespoon chia seeds

- 1 teaspoon lime juice

- Ice cubes (optional)

Prep Time: 7 mins

Total Time: 7 mins

Servings: 1

Nutrition Facts (per serving):

- Calories: 220

- Protein: 5g

- Carbohydrates: 35g

- Fat: 10g

- Fiber: 8g

Directions:

1. In a blender, combine pineapple chunks, coconut milk, shredded coconut, banana, chia seeds, and lime juice.

2. Blend until smooth and transport yourself to a tropical paradise.

3. Add ice cubes if desired and blend again.

4. Pour into a glass and savor the tropical flavors of this pineapple coconut paradise smoothie.

APPETIZER RECIPES

Zesty Guacamole with Veggie Sticks

Ingredients:

- 2 ripe avocados, mashed
- 1 medium tomato, diced
- 1/4 cup red onion, finely chopped
- 1/4 cup cilantro, chopped
- 1 clove garlic, minced
- 1 lime, juiced
- Salt and pepper to taste
- Assorted vegetable sticks (carrots, cucumber, bell peppers) for dipping

Prep Time: 10 mins

Total Time: 10 mins

Servings: 4

Nutrition Facts (per serving):

- Calories: 120
- Protein: 2g

- Carbohydrates: 10g

- Fat: 9g

- Fiber: 6g

Directions:

1. In a bowl, combine mashed avocados, diced tomato, chopped red onion, cilantro, minced garlic, and lime juice.

2. Season with salt and pepper to taste.

3. Mix well and refrigerate for at least 30 minutes to enhance flavors.

4. Serve with assorted vegetable sticks for a refreshing and nutritious appetizer.

Protein-Packed Hummus Platter

Ingredients:

- 1 can (15 oz) chickpeas, drained and rinsed

- 1/4 cup tahini

- 1/4 cup olive oil

- 1 clove garlic, minced

- 1 lemon, juiced

- Salt and cumin to taste

- Assorted whole-grain crackers and cucumber slices for serving

Prep Time: 15 mins

Total Time: 15 mins

Servings: 6

Nutrition Facts (per serving):

- Calories: 180

- Protein: 7g

- Carbohydrates: 15g

- Fat: 11g

- Fiber: 5g

Directions:

1. In a food processor, combine chickpeas, tahini, olive oil, minced garlic, lemon juice, salt, and cumin.

2. Blend until smooth and creamy, adding water if needed to achieve desired consistency.

3. Transfer hummus to a serving bowl and drizzle with olive oil.

4. Serve with whole-grain crackers and cucumber slices for a protein-packed appetizer.

Savory Stuffed Mushrooms

Ingredients:

- 12 large mushrooms, stems removed and finely chopped

- 1/2 cup breadcrumbs (whole grain)

- 1/4 cup Parmesan cheese, grated

- 2 tablespoons olive oil

- 2 cloves garlic, minced

- 1/4 cup fresh parsley, chopped

- Salt and pepper to taste

Prep Time: 20 mins

Total Time: 35 mins

Servings: 4

Nutrition Facts (per serving):

- Calories: 130

- Protein: 5g

- Carbohydrates: 10g

- Fat: 8g

- Fiber: 2g

Directions:

1. Preheat oven to 375°F (190°C).

2. In a bowl, combine chopped mushroom stems, breadcrumbs, Parmesan cheese, olive oil, minced garlic, fresh parsley, salt, and pepper.

3. Spoon the mixture into the mushroom caps.

4. Place stuffed mushrooms on a baking sheet and bake for 15-20 minutes or until golden brown.

5. Serve warm as a savory and satisfying appetizer.

Smoked Salmon Cucumber Bites

Ingredients:

- 1 English cucumber, sliced

- 4 oz smoked salmon, cut into small pieces

- 1/4 cup cream cheese

- 1 tablespoon fresh dill, chopped

- 1 teaspoon capers (optional)

Prep Time: 15 mins

Total Time: 15 mins

Servings: 4

Nutrition Facts (per serving):

- Calories: 90

- Protein: 8g

- Carbohydrates: 3g

- Fat: 5g

- Fiber: 1g

Directions:

1. Arrange cucumber slices on a serving platter.

2. Spread a thin layer of cream cheese on each cucumber slice.

3. Top with smoked salmon pieces and sprinkle fresh dill.

4. Garnish with capers if desired.

5. Serve these elegant and flavourful bites as a light appetizer.

Roasted Red Pepper and White Bean Dip

Ingredients:

- 1 can (15 oz) white beans, drained and rinsed

- 1/2 cup roasted red peppers, drained

- 2 tablespoons olive oil

- 1 clove garlic, minced

- 1 tablespoon lemon juice

- Salt and paprika to taste

- Whole-grain pita bread or vegetable sticks for dipping

Prep Time: 10 mins

Total Time: 20 mins

Servings: 4

Nutrition Facts (per serving):

- Calories: 120

- Protein: 5g

- Carbohydrates: 16g

- Fat: 5g

- Fiber: 4g

Directions:

1. In a food processor, combine white beans, roasted red peppers, olive oil, minced garlic, lemon juice, salt, and paprika.

2. Blend until smooth and creamy.

3. Transfer the dip to a serving bowl.

4. Serve with whole-grain pita bread or vegetable sticks for a flavourful and satisfying appetizer.

Crispy Baked Kale Chips

Ingredients:

- 1 bunch kale, stems removed and torn into bite-sized pieces

- 1 tablespoon olive oil

- 1/2 teaspoon sea salt

- 1/4 teaspoon garlic powder

- 1/4 teaspoon paprika (optional)

Prep Time: 10 mins

Total Time: 20 mins

Servings: 4

Nutrition Facts (per serving):

- Calories: 50

- Protein: 2g

- Carbohydrates: 5g

- Fat: 3g

- Fiber: 2g

Directions:

1. Preheat the oven to 350°F (175°C).

2. In a bowl, toss kale pieces with olive oil, sea salt, garlic powder, and paprika.

3. Spread the kale on a baking sheet in a single layer.

4. Bake for 10-15 minutes or until crispy, turning once halfway through.

5. Allow to cool before serving as a nutritious and crunchy snack.

Mango Salsa with Baked Pita Chips

Ingredients:

- 1 ripe mango, diced

- 1/2 red onion, finely chopped

- 1/4 cup fresh cilantro, chopped

- 1 jalapeño, seeded and minced

- 1 lime, juiced

- Salt to taste

- Whole-grain pita bread, cut into wedges for baking

Prep Time: 15 mins

Total Time: 25 mins

Servings: 4

Nutrition Facts (per serving):

- Calories: 90

- Protein: 2g

- Carbohydrates: 20g

- Fat: 1g

- Fiber: 3g

Directions:

1. Preheat the oven to 375°F (190°C).

2. In a bowl, combine diced mango, chopped red onion, cilantro, minced jalapeño, lime juice, and salt.

3. Arrange pita wedges on a baking sheet and bake for 8-10 minutes or until golden and crisp.

4. Serve the mango salsa with baked pita chips for a refreshing and fruity appetizer.

Greek Yogurt Dip with Vegetable Sticks

Ingredients:

- 1 cup Greek yogurt

- 1 tablespoon fresh dill, chopped

- 1 tablespoon lemon juice

- 1 clove garlic, minced

- Salt and pepper to taste

- Assorted vegetable sticks (carrots, cucumber, bell peppers) for dipping

Prep Time: 10 mins

Total Time: 10 mins

Servings: 4

Nutrition Facts (per serving):

- Calories: 60

- Protein: 6g

- Carbohydrates: 5g

- Fat: 2g

- Fiber: 1g

Directions:

1. In a bowl, combine Greek yogurt, chopped fresh dill, lemon juice, minced garlic, salt, and pepper.

2. Mix well until smooth and creamy.

3. Refrigerate for at least 30 minutes before serving.

4. Serve with assorted vegetable sticks for a protein-rich and satisfying dip.

Quinoa-Stuffed Bell Peppers

Ingredients:

- 4 bell peppers, halved and seeds removed

- 1 cup cooked quinoa

- 1 can (15 oz) black beans, drained and rinsed

- 1 cup corn kernels

- 1 cup cherry tomatoes, halved

- 1/4 cup fresh cilantro, chopped

- 1 teaspoon cumin

- Salt and pepper to taste

Prep Time: 20 mins

Total Time: 45 mins

Servings: 4

Nutrition Facts (per serving):

- Calories: 180

- Protein: 8g

- Carbohydrates: 35g

- Fat: 2g

- Fiber: 7g

Directions:

1. Preheat the oven to 375°F (190°C).

2. In a bowl, combine cooked quinoa, black beans, corn kernels, cherry tomatoes, chopped cilantro, cumin, salt, and pepper.

3. Fill each bell pepper half with the quinoa mixture.

4. Bake for 25-30 minutes or until peppers are tender.

5. Serve these quinoa-stuffed bell peppers as a wholesome and flavourful appetizer.

Cucumber and Hummus Roll-Ups

Ingredients:

- 1 large cucumber, thinly sliced lengthwise

- 1/2 cup hummus

- 1/4 cup cherry tomatoes, halved

- 1/4 cup Kalamata olives, sliced

- 2 tablespoons crumbled feta cheese

- Fresh mint leaves for garnish

Prep Time: 15 mins

Total Time: 15 mins

Servings: 4

Nutrition Facts (per serving):

- Calories: 80

- Protein: 3g

- Carbohydrates: 8g

- Fat: 5g

- Fiber: 2g

Directions:

1. Lay cucumber slices flat and spread a thin layer of hummus on each slice.

2. Place cherry tomatoes, Kalamata olives, and crumbled feta along the length of each slice.

3. Roll up the cucumber slices and secure them with toothpicks.

4. Garnish with fresh mint leaves before serving these light and tasty roll-ups.

14-DAY MEAL PLAN

Day 1:

- *Breakfast:* Quinoa Breakfast Bowl

- *Lunch:* Protein-Packed Hummus Platter

- *Dinner:* Quinoa-Stuffed Bell Peppers

Day 2:

- *Breakfast:* Avocado Toast with Poached Egg

- *Lunch:* Crispy Baked Kale Chips

- *Dinner:* Zesty Guacamole with Veggie Sticks

Day 3:

- *Breakfast:* Cottage Cheese and Fruit Bowl

- *Lunch:* Greek Yogurt Dip with Vegetable Sticks

- *Dinner:* Roasted Red Pepper and White Bean Dip

Day 4:

- *Breakfast:* Spinach and Mushroom Omelette

- *Lunch:* Mango Salsa with Baked Pita Chips

- *Dinner:* Cucumber and Hummus Roll-Ups

Day 5:

- *Breakfast:* Quinoa Breakfast Bowl

- *Lunch:* Savory Stuffed Mushrooms

- *Dinner:* Easy Fried Rice

Day 6:

- *Breakfast:* Avocado Toast with Poached Egg

- *Lunch:* Crispy Baked Kale Chips

- *Dinner:* Cottage Cheese and Fruit Bowl

Day 7:

- *Breakfast:* Quinoa Breakfast Bowl

- *Lunch:* Greek Yogurt Dip with Vegetable Sticks

- *Dinner:* Zesty Guacamole with Veggie Sticks

Day 8:

- *Breakfast:* Spinach and Mushroom Omelette

- *Lunch:* Protein-Packed Hummus Platter

- *Dinner:* Quinoa-Stuffed Bell Peppers

Day 9:

- *Breakfast:* Cottage Cheese and Fruit Bowl

- *Lunch:* Mango Salsa with Baked Pita Chips

- *Dinner:* Roasted Red Pepper and White Bean Dip

Day 10:

- ***Breakfast:*** Avocado Toast with Poached Egg

- ***Lunch:*** Crispy Baked Kale Chips

- ***Dinner:*** Cucumber and Hummus Roll-Ups

Day 11:

- ***Breakfast:*** Quinoa Breakfast Bowl

- ***Lunch:*** Savory Stuffed Mushrooms

- ***Dinner:*** Easy Fried Rice

Day 12:

- ***Breakfast:*** Cottage Cheese and Fruit Bowl

- ***Lunch:*** Protein-Packed Hummus Platter

- ***Dinner:*** Quinoa-stuffed Bell Peppers

Day 13:

- ***Breakfast:*** Avocado Toast with Poached Egg

- ***Lunch:*** Mango Salsa with Baked Pita Chips

- ***Dinner:*** Zesty Guacamole with Veggie Sticks

Day 14:

- ***Breakfast:*** Spinach and Mushroom Omelette

- ***Lunch:*** Greek Yogurt Dip with Vegetable Sticks

- ***Dinner:*** Roasted Red Pepper and White Bean Dip

CONCLUSION

In conclusion, the "LYMPHEDEMA DIET COOKBOOK FOR SENIORS" offers a holistic approach to managing lymphedema through nutrition and lifestyle choices. Understanding lymphedema as a chronic condition characterized by fluid retention, the cookbook delves into the specifics of how this condition affects seniors.

The book emphasizes the importance of adopting a Lymphedema Diet, outlining key principles that focus on reducing inflammation, supporting the lymphatic system, and maintaining an overall healthy lifestyle. Central to this approach is the incorporation of nutrient-rich recipes designed with seniors in mind.

Recognizing the vital role of proper nutrition for seniors, the cookbook underscores the significance of a well-balanced diet in managing lymphedema symptoms. The recipes provided are not only delicious but also tailored to meet the nutritional needs of seniors, addressing concerns such as protein intake, fiber content, and overall caloric requirements.

Hydration emerges as a critical component in lymphedema management, with the cookbook extensively discussing the role of proper fluid balance. Practical tips for seniors on staying well-hydrated are highlighted, promoting overall health and aiding in the management of lymphatic congestion.

The incorporation of gentle exercises is presented as a complementary strategy, recognizing that physical activity contributes to improved lymphatic circulation. Additionally, stress management and relaxation techniques are explored as essential elements in promoting overall well-being, acknowledging the interconnectedness of mental and physical health.

To make the transition into a lymphedema-friendly diet seamless, the cookbook provides a variety of recipes, ranging from nutritious breakfast options like the Quinoa Breakfast Bowl to satisfying lunch and dinner choices such as the Quinoa-Stuffed Bell Peppers. Snacks, appetizers, and desserts are also included, ensuring a diverse and enjoyable culinary experience.

9 798320 124797